Intermittent Fasting:

An Easy Way to Lose Weight, Cleanse Your Body, Increase Energy Levels & Reduce Inflammation

Karen Dixon
© **April 2020**

Notarial Notes

The contents presented herein constitute the rights of the First Amendment. All information states to be truthful, accurate, reliable, and consistent. Any liability, by way of inattention or otherwise, to any use or abuse of any policies, processes, or directions contained within, is the sole discretion and responsibility of the recipient reader.

The presentation of the entire information is without a contract or any form of guarantees or assurances. Both author and publisher shall be, in no case, held liable for any fraud or fraudulent misrepresentations, monetary losses, damages, and liabilities—indirect or consequential—arising from event/s beyond reasonable control or relatively set out in this book.

Therefore, any information hereupon solely offers for educational purposes only, and as such, universal. It does not intend to be a diagnosis, prescription, or treatment for any diseases.

The Food and Drug Administration has not evaluated the statements in the book. If advice is necessary, consult a qualified professional for further questions concerning specific or critical matters on the subject.

The trademarks used herein are without any consent. Thus, the publication of the trademark is without any permission or backing by the trademark owner/s.

All trademarks/brands mentioned are for clarification purposes only and owned by the owners themselves not affiliated with the author or publisher.

TABLE OF CONTENTS

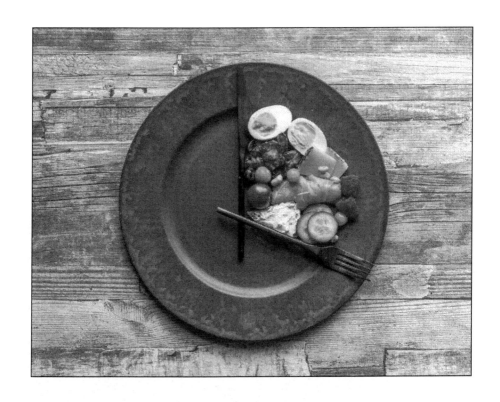

Introduction

Fasting is an old custom practiced by various nationalities and cultures in early times. Beneficial intermittent fasts for solving problems with excessive fat were studied as early as 1915. This captured the attention of the medical world in the mid-1900s after Bloom and company made a viable report. Intermittent fasts, also known as IF, were in the range of 1 to 14 days in these studies.

This interest started being shared in bulletins, which reminded people to be aware and careful about the use of intermittent fasting without advice from a medical professional.

The latest kind of intermittent fasting is also known as the 5:2 Diet which started in Britain several years ago.

There is a variety of intermittent fasting which can be found in religious traditions all over the globe. Examples of religious fasting include Vrata, Ramadan, Christian Fasting, and many more. Some religious fasting customs only require staying away from certain foods, while others, such as Yom Kippur, require not eating food for a brief period and might result in unnoticeable effects on a person's BMI.

In Buddhism, skipping a meal is considered part of the enhancement of knowledge of the monks, who skip meals regularly for more than 12 hours a day. This regular skipping of meals may be executed by any persons that are undergoing the eight principles.

During Muslim fasting, which is relatively similar to intermittent fasting and includes depriving oneself of food or drink for several hours, one must omit the consumption of food up until sunrise and after sunset.

A study on the health of Muslims during their fasting period show a tremendous loss in weight during said period of up to 1.5 kg, but this weight came back approximately after 14 days when the fasting ended.

To sum it up, the holy feast gives a way to lose weight, but well-built and steady lifestyle changes are crucial to achieve permanent weight loss. There is a study that has proven that the same traits exist in Ramadan fasting and eating with a time constraint, with the primary difference being the deprivation of drinking liquids with Muslim fasting. Some of the bad effects of Muslim fasting comprise elevated hazards of hypoglycemia in people with diabetes and imbalanced levels of some nutrients.

The prevention of consuming liquids while in the fasting stage of Muslim fasting is risky for women that are pregnant because it is linked to the dangers of inducing labor and can be the main cause of gestational diabetes, although it isn't shown to have an effect on the child's weight.

Chapter 1: Fundamentals of Intermittent Fasting

Intermittent fasting is a food consumption methodology that alternates between the limitation of calorie consumption or skipping meals and the usual food consumption during a certain time period. There are various kinds of intermittent fasting routines, such as the 5:2 diet, and many more. The most famous type of intermittent fasting is the 16:8 method, which comprises eating during an 8-hour timeframe before skipping meals for 16 hours.

Weight loss is the most common factor for individuals to attempt intermittent fasting. By allowing you to consume fewer meals, intermittent fasting can result in an immediate decrease in calorie intake.

Furthermore, intermittent fasting alters hormone levels to help in losing weight. In addition to lessening insulin levels and elevating human growth hormone (HGH) levels, it increases the expulsion of the fat reduction hormone. Because of these alterations in hormones, temporary fasting may elevate your metabolic rate by a maximum of 14%. As a result of you consuming less and reducing your calorie intake, intermittent fasting causes weight reduction by altering both parts of the calorie equation.

Researchers have found that intermittent fasting can be a strong weight reduction tool. It is known that this consuming pattern can result in a 3 to 8 percent weight loss over 1 to 6 months, which is a huge amount if compared to a lot of weight reduction research. Individuals who reduced 4 to 7 percent of their waistline, also showed a huge reduction of dangerous belly fat that accumulates around your organs and results in illnesses.

Intermittent fasting causes less muscle loss than the more conventional technique of general limiting of one's calorie intake. However, it is important to take into consideration that the primary factor for its triumph is that intermittent fasting encourages you to consume fewer calories. If you consume massive amounts of food when you do eat, you may not lose any weight at all.

Intermittent fasting is primarily utilized as a weight reduction routine. But it is proven it may also be advantageous to one's health in various ways.

For instance, intermittent fasting has been shown to lessen inflammation and enhance brain responsiveness and glucose levels. This is why intermittent fasting is an eating pattern that comprises cycling between the stages in which you normally eat or skip meals.

When you skip meals, a lot of things can occur in your body, particularly on the level of hormones and cells. For example, your body calibrates hormone levels to allow easy access to your storage of body fat. Your cells also start crucial fixing processes and alter the structure of genes.

Here are some alterations that happen in your body when you skip meals:

- **Human Growth Hormone (HGH):** The human growth hormone significantly increases, rising to at least 5 times more than the standard amount. This is beneficial for losing weight and gaining muscle mass.

- **Insulin:** Sensitivity to insulin enhances and insulin levels decrease significantly. Decreasing insulin levels transform body fat storage to make it accessible.

- **Cellular Repair:** When you skip meals, your cells start cellular fixing processes. This includes autophagy, where cells take in good proteins and expel bad proteins that accumulate inside cells.

- **Gene Expression:** There are alterations in the usage of genes linked to long lifespan and security against disease.

These alterations in hormone levels, cell usage, and gene characteristics are some of the main health advantages of intermittent fasting. When you skip meals, HGH levels rise and insulin levels decrease. Your body's cells alter the characteristics of genes and start crucial cellular fixation processes.

Chapter 2: Techniques for Intermittent Fasting

Intermittent fasting is an example of fasting and eating over a specific time span, and it isn't characterized by specific types of foods. It is suggested that you consume food during your eating phase.

Intermittent fasting can be used sometimes or frequently to suit your needs. You may even prefer to mix constantly, doing it every day or opting for a monthly or yearly basis. The sum total of strategies that exist have been shown to be powerful, but through research and experimentation, you will find the one that suits you best.

To give you the power to choose, here's a run-through of the different sorts of intermittent fasting.

Every Day Fasting or Time-Restricted Eating

This is a good and practical strategy for fasting that can be integrated into your daily life. With the approach in question, you limit eating to 4 to 11-hours, while fasting for 13–20 hours. Basically, you drag out your last meal fast by postponing your initial meal of the day, stop consuming foods before the day starts or both. This kind of fasting is usually implemented continuously, but a few people devote all their time to it, depending on their schedule.

The 16:8 Method: Fast for 16 Hours Every Day

This method includes fasting each day for 14-16 hours and limiting your "eating phase" to 8-10 hours. Inside the eating phase, you can fit in 2, 3, or more meals. This strategy is also called the Leangains routine. Following this approach to fasting can be the same as not having anything after your last meal and skipping breakfast the next day.

In the case that you finish your last eating phase at 8 p.m. and don't eat until 12 noon the following day, at that specific time you are already skipping eating for 16 hours between meals.

It is more advisable for women because it is 14-15 hours of fasting which is better as they are more responsive to short-paced fasting.

For those who are attempting to lose weight, it can be difficult to become acclimated to skipping breakfast from the outset since their body is most likely to crave breakfast upon waking up. However, several breakfast enthusiasts eat tremendously along with said phase.

You can drink liquids (non-caloric) during the skipping meals phase, and this can help lessen hunger levels. It is mandatory to consume solid foods during your eating phase. This won't work if you eat portions of non-nutritious foods or if you exceed your allowed measures of calories.

People can consider this a usual approach to intermittent fasting. I also believe it myself and find it completely easy to follow. I eat a low-carb diet, so my hunger is managed fairly well. I don't feel hungry until around 1 p.m. onwards. This is why I eat my last supper around 6-9 p.m., so as a result, I fast for approximately 16-19 hours.

To conclude, the 16:8 strategy includes day to day fasts of 16 hours for men and 14-15 hours for women. Every day, you lessen your food consumption to an 8-10 hour "eating phase" where you can fit in 2-3 or more healthy meals.

The 20:4 Method: Fast for 20 Hours Every Day

The 20:4 approach is a kind of intermittent fasting that is reliant upon a 20-hour fast, with a 4-hour eating window. For the most part, you can consume food in whatever amount you might want during the 4-hour gap; however, it is hard to digest an excessive number of calories during such a short period of time.

The 4-hour eating window usually happens at night but can occur in any part of the day that suits you. For example, you can eat two dinners somewhere in the span of 2 p.m. and 6 p.m., and fast for approximately 20 hours.

This would be appropriate for people who are certain about intermittent fasting, are occupied during the day because they work and don't have the chance to consume foods, don't feel hungry during the day, or find that eating makes them less productive and drowsy.

This technique can be implemented for unique events regardless of whether you're taking off for a dinner or going to devour a delectable meal with loved ones.

Extended Fasts

These are usually not done on a daily basis but intermittently. These variations of fasts are great for individuals who have already determined that they can't focus on a daily fast; however, they might want to add it into their weekly, monthly, or yearly timetable.

If you already practice restraint eating, you might consider extensive fasting during the time to upgrade your ketosis to the next level.

The 5:2 Diet: Fast for 2 Days out of Every Week

This routine comprises of consuming foods for 5 days of the week while lowering calories down to 500-600 on two days of the week. This eating routine is known as the "Fast Eating Regimen" and was formulated by Michael Mosley. In the fasting phase, it is recommended that women consume at most 500 calories and men 600 calories at most.

Moreover, you may eat properly on all days with the exception of Mondays and Thursdays (for example), where you eat 2 low-calorie meals (250 calories for each meal for women, and 300 for men).

As doubters continuously bring up, there is no medical proof for the 5:2 eating routine itself, yet there are a lot of notable advantages of intermittent fasting.

So, the 5:2 eating routine includes eating 500-600 calories for two days of the week but consuming foods daily on the other 5 days.

Eat-Stop-Eat: Do a 24-Hour Quick Fast

This includes a 24-hour quick fast a few times every week. This way of eating has been mainstream for several years in the fitness world. By fasting from one meal, most probably the first meal of a day, to the last meal continuously this adds up to a 24-hour fast.

If you finished the last meal by Monday at 7 p.m., and haven't eaten anything until the last meal the following day at 7 p.m., at that specific time you've done an entire 24-hour fast. You refrain from eating meals from the first meal to the first meal or the second meal to the second meal. The final product is the same.

Non-caloric liquid drinks can be consumed during the fasting phase. If you are doing this to get fitter and healthier, then it is important that you typically eat during the eating time frames. As in, eat the same amount of foods as though you have not been fasting.

The issue with this technique is that an entire 24-hour quick fast can be difficult for some people. The way you don't have to put everything on the line immediately is to begin with 14-16 hours and continuing from that point onward is fine.

It is proven that the initial part of the fasting phase is simple; however, I realized that whenever I was doing it, I became voraciously ravenous when eating. I expected to apply genuine discipline in order to complete the full 24-hours because a lack of control when it comes to food consumption might result in failure.

To conclude, this routine is an intermittent fasting program that requires you to perform a few 24-hour fasts every week.

36-Hour Fasting

This is a unique form of the 24-hour fast. You will have to consume foods at the very beginning, fast for the sum of day two, and have breakfast on day three. This kind of fasting can assist in your transition into ketosis or push you into a better scenario of ketosis. This should be possible to do occasionally or as frequently as once every 7 days, 30 days, or more.

Alternate Day Fasting: Fast Every Other Day

This kind of fasting encourages you to skip meals every other day, but there are a few unique adaptations of this. Some of those routines allow the intake of approximately 500 calories during the fasting phase. Many consider that alternate day fasting demonstrates the medical advantages of intermittent fasting when utilized properly. A full fast that is done every other day is not for the faint-hearted because it is too hardcore, so I would not recommend this to individuals who are just trying to start intermittent fasting.

With this routine, you will be going to sleep with the feeling of hunger a few times each week, which is not desirable and advisable for the long-term. This approach involves skipping meals every other day, either by not eating anything or just eating a few calories.

Unconstrained Fasting

This is one approach that I would recommend for any person who is hesitant about intermittent fasting or feels overpowered by going into unadvisable fasting times.

This is a delicate approach to intermittent fasting, which is driven by your way of life and body. It is perfect for people who prefer not to feel limited or get incapacitated if they don't meet the criteria of their food consumption routine.

With this approach, you skip meals if you don't feel hungry or are too busy to remember eating. Cooking and food consumption takes up a lot of time. Grasping the reasons why you eat will give you the advantage to take different steps, such as combining dinner with some recreational activities that are also beneficial for your health, like brisk walking or yoga. Mind conditioning is a successful method to recondition the prevalent view that we have to eat three full meals per day.

By lowering your intake of calories, all of these techniques should result in weight loss as long as you do not consume more than the normal amount of foods during your eating period.

A lot of individuals have recognized the 16:8 technique as the most noncomplex, easy to maintain and be consistent with technique. It is also the most famous technique among all.

No matter what intermittent fasting approach you choose to follow, keep in mind, the calories and the quality of foods are crucial and shouldn't be ignored. There are times that people can side-line food quality or over enjoy in calories as they utilize intermittent fasting as a resort to enhance their well-being. Over the long term, this won't be viable, and your wellness will be undermined.

Have a great time and try the different sorts of intermittent fasting to see which one you like best.

Chapter 3: Intermittent Fasting and Autophagy

Normally, autophagy is a critical piece of cell work, in which "flawed" cells (for example, ones that may somehow lead to ailment), dead, or worn-out cells are dismantled to make new cells.

A few people have found autophagy helps diminish ailment, lessens irritation, and reinforces the immune system to become stronger. Autophagy has some links to mental instability and schizophrenia. In some people, it's feasible that autophagy could be utilized to lengthen their life span, despite the minimal studies made to prove it.

Scientists are very curious about the possibility that fasting-prompted autophagy can be a potential cause for tumor growth, despite the fact that it has a lot of benefits. Many believe that when the treatment of malignant growth is supplemented by fasting, if you include customary medication, similar to chemotherapy, the results of recovery and healing can be really devastating, but that's not the case for some.

Then again, you should consider that autophagy can have the contrary impact, by making tumors increasingly impervious to radiation. Furthermore, autophagy has both positive and negative implications for cancer, and this has been shown by evidence about whether or how autophagy limitation can be utilized in cancer removal.

It is known that women who have recovered from cancer found that those who fasted for over 13 hours daily had lower chances of their cancer coming back. A few different studies are underway — on the results of fasting on lung cancer, prostate disease, glioblastoma, and breast and ovarian tumors — the results of which are all positive because of the manifestations autophagy is showing in responding to those kinds of diseases.

People are worried that a lot of fasting-prompted weight reduction could be risky, especially for individuals diagnosed with cancer. So, when autophagy occurs, is it occurring all over one's body?

Fundamentally, with a remarkable exemption: fasting seems to actuate autophagy in many organs (like the liver, muscles, and pancreas). Are there any benefits of autophagy that sound unrealistic, and are there reasons why you are reluctant about trying it?

All things considered, though it may sound unrealistic — this unfathomably simple approach to fixing health issues — I particularly like the obscure thought that autophagy could be useful for the buildup of scales for skin infections like psoriasis. There is also hearsay about people who lost massive weight by means of skipping meals but did not need to undergo medical methods that are needed to fix their saggy skin after losing a lot of weight.

Research on fasting-prompted autophagy specifically, in people, is prevalent. There is a study on autophagy and human sickness abridged autophagy as being related to an expanding number of diseases, from bacterial and viral contaminations to cancers, and more as of late in neurodegenerative and other age-related infections.

Autophagy has been known to be beneficial and not beneficial all at the same time due to its power to provide advantages to human health or even damage. Skipping meals, as a rule, can add to the growth of gallstones, which can grow when bile that is put away in the gallbladder solidifies into stone-like tissue. It is also not recommended for people who are underweight, pregnant women, toddlers, and others with specialized conditions.

Could fasting to actuate autophagy be depicted as an eating disorder? Not characteristically, but unnecessary fasting to instigate autophagy could actually result in anorexia. Lots of people fast because of the benefit of controlling their weight; however, there are more benefits including combating infection, muscle maintenance, and mental health improvement.

Would you be able to fast to trigger autophagy to occur every now and then? There are no accurate measures on that, but experts say that all-inclusive fasting for autophagy — like going for 36, 48, or even 72 hours without consuming foods — is something that serious individuals must do 2 or 3 times each year, and with a supervision of an expert.

Is there a way to know whether autophagy is going on in your body? Is there a way to quantify it? Determining autophagy in people or knowing the "autophagic motion" is unreliable when it includes the rising and falling proportions of certain small portions of proteins (like the protein LC3 and its variations).

There's nothing like an "autophagometer," for example, and a recent report noticed that it's somehow hard to screen autophagy suitably in people. However, you can weigh things like glucose and ketones, which are influenced by fasting.

Chapter 4: Intermittent Fasting and Keto Diet

The keto diet is a high-fat, low carbohydrate diet. Carbohydrates are usually decreased to less than 50 g per day, which pushes your body to be dependent on fats, as a substitute for glucose, as its primary energy supply.

In this metabolic process, also called ketosis, your body crushes fats to create substances known as ketones that use as a substitute fuel supply.

This diet is a crucial step to losing weight, but it has more advantages than just that. It has also been utilized for a lot of years to cure epilepsy and has been found to be beneficial for other neurological disorders.

For instance, the keto diet may improve mental health in individuals with Alzheimer's disease. Furthermore, it may lessen blood sugar levels, enhance insulin resistance, and decrease heart disease risks like triglyceride levels.

If you take part in a ketogenic diet while doing intermittent fasting as well, it could give you the following advantages.

Intermittent fasting may help your body obtain ketosis faster than just doing a keto diet. The primary reason behind this is your body, when fasting, retains its energy equilibrium by changing its fuel supply from carbohydrates to fats – the precise aim of the keto diet. In fasting, insulin levels and glycogen storage decrease, causing your body to logically initiate using fat for fuel, thereby decreasing your storage of fat.

For individuals who struggle to obtain ketosis while on a keto diet, supplementing it with intermittent fasting may initiate this process.

Mixing the keto diet and intermittent fasting can help you reduce more fat than by solely doing a keto diet. This is because intermittent fasting accelerates your metabolism by initiating thermogenesis, or the production of heat in your body, it may, the usage of fat storage. Intermittent fasting can extensively and safely reduce extra body fat. In an 8-week study in 34 males, those who implemented the 16:8 routine of intermittent fasting dropped at least 14% more body fat than those who practiced a standard eating regimen.

Likewise, there are people who have proven that by implementing intermittent fasting they deduct an average of 7 lbs. more fat mass than those who follow extremely low-calorie diets.

Additionally, intermittent fasting may retain muscle mass during weight reduction and enhance energy levels, which may be beneficial for individuals who are practicing a keto diet, who are aiming to enhance their performance in sports and reduce body fat. Furthermore, it is proven that intermittent fasting can lessen the feeling of hunger and replace it with the feeling of being full, which might be beneficial for losing weight.

Mixing intermittent fasting with a keto diet may help you reach ketosis much quicker and reduce more body fat than by solely relying on a keto diet.

Mixing a keto diet with intermittent fasting is safe for most individuals. However, pregnant or breastfeeding women and individuals who are experiencing or have experienced eating disorders in the past should seek professional medical advice before attempting to do intermittent fasting.

Individuals with health issues, such as diabetes or heart ailments, should seek professional help prior to doing intermittent fasting while on the keto diet.

Though many individuals may consider combining the methods beneficial, it's crucial to remember that it might not function for everyone. Some may find that skipping meals on the keto diet is really hard, or they may experience bad effects, such as binge eating during the non-fasting period, uneasiness, and weariness.

Keep in mind that intermittent fasting is not required to obtain ketosis, even though it can be utilized as a way to achieve ketosis in a much faster way.

Simply implementing a healthy keto diet is sufficient for anyone searching to enhance their health by lowering their carb intake. Though continuous intermittent fasting and ketogenic dieting may improve each other's efficiency, it's not necessary to mix both. Depending upon your health aspirations, you may select one over its counterpart.

It is suggested to try out things and check if it is feasible in order to be certain that it will give you the best results. However, with any big lifestyle transformation, it is recommended to talk to your healthcare provider beforehand.

Chapter 5: Intermittent Fasting for Women

Pregnancy and Intermittent Fasting

Is it OK for you to do intermittent fasting while pregnant? As was said earlier, first address your primary care physician before rolling out any delicate improvements to your eating routine and exercise caution.

There is not a large amount of research to give educated suggestions as to whether there are sure or negative impacts on the pregnancy. There are no studies that looked at intermittent fasting over the entire length of pregnancy.

A large number of studies that look at pregnant women and fasting focus on the Islamic custom of Ramadan, which lasts around 30 days. During that period, individuals fast from sunup to sundown. While pregnant and breastfeeding moms are in fact freed from fasting, some still carry on with fasting.

There is a study conducted on a group of women which suggests that those who fasted during Ramadan experienced large changes in their glucose, insulin, and triglyceride levels, just like the other studies have found. The weight of their children during labor was similar to the infants of women who had not fasted.

A later study suggests these results and says that fasting for Ramadan doesn't affect childbirth. Aside from that, there was no relationship between fasting and birth. Just like what our forefathers believed in the past; however, experts presume that more studies are required on fasting and its potential risk and impact on health.

One thing we know is that pregnancy is the point at which you have to focus on:

- Helping your child put on weight
- Providing sustenance to help with mind and body improvement
- Developing maternal fat stores if you want to breastfeed

Significantly changing dietary patterns may inflict a lack of nutrients and other medical problems for both you and your child. Fasting might also change hormone levels.

Also, know that intermittent fasting and pregnancy manage birth weight. There is such a large number of other potential effects that haven't been examined — for instance, the dangers, later on, affecting kids whose moms did intermittent fasting while pregnant, for instance.

Most importantly, the way fasting affects your body and pregnancy is variable and inconsistent in relation to how it may affect another person. Experts suggest that you work with your doctor to build up some preparation for the weight increase that will happen, and all preparations should be based on your weight (BMI) and overall wellness.

For women with BMIs in the 18.5 to 24.9 range, this usually includes being up somewhere in the measure of 25 and 35 pounds eating a fair eating regimen of wholefoods and drinking a lot of water. Those with more weight may need to control increase under the direction of an expert with cautious surveillance of their child's development.

Imagine a scenario if a woman practiced intermittent fasting before pregnancy. This may seem over exaggerated, but it is not. Talk to your doctor if you're, as of now, planning to fast to see what will work for you. It may be alright for you to keep fasting, just not precisely as you might have so far. Make sure to tell your primary care physician your whole history with intermittent fasting, as well as your goals in continuing with it during pregnancy.

While the long-term implications aren't absolutely clear, scientists examined women fasting for Ramadan and how it influenced things like fetal development. At the point when ladies had low glucose levels from fasting, it took them a usually longer amount of time to distinguish fetal developments.

The low reappearance of fetal developments is usually determined as a notice sign you must pay attention to, specifically, as you draw nearer to your due date. Your infant should make around 10 developments inside an hour to 2, and you will already feel improvements inside half an hour.

With confining eating to specific windows or days, it may be hard to get the ideal measure of food when you are eating. This might be problematic if your child is pulling from your food storage too.

The issues like low iron are very common for pregnant women. What's more, when a child doesn't get enough iron — especially in the third trimester — they may be at increased risk of getting ill before their first birthday. This is alarming but fortunately getting good foods causes these risks to decrease.

To prevent weight increase consistently in a healthy way, most women should target to consume 300 extra kcals every day. That is a little extra — like a glass of skim milk and a huge piece of a sandwich — yet absolutely not the "eating for two" you may have heard before you got pregnant.

Exercise is another piece of the circumstance. You may feel cruddy — particularly in the first trimester — however, moving your body may lower your hazard of gestational diabetes, help to increase your physical performance, and lessen your chances of needing a cesarean.

If you've exercised before pregnancy, it will be truly amazing! Ask whether you have to regulate your daily schedule and continue onward. In case you're new to workouts, focus on getting around 30 minutes every day of light exercises, such as strolling, swimming, or cycling.

Shouldn't something be said about intermittent fasting and attempting to get pregnant? At the moment, for some entirely cool news, studies show there's a "commonly useful" tie between the way of eating and fertility. Intermittent fasting may have some influence on fertility in women with polycystic ovary disorder (PCOS). In one ongoing study, women with weight and PCOS who skipped meals usually saw an expansion in their hormonal levels, which is crucial for aiding in ovulation.

Other data suggest that weight reduction of 5 to 10 percent may help with reproduction. Since intermittent fasting may help here, just as with insulin opposition and other medical problems, it's plausible that fasting may "progress" the richness and soundness of the human body.

It's not a smart idea to dive into fasting during pregnancy — particularly if you haven't tried it before. Luckily pregnancy doesn't keep going forever, and you can attempt this methodology for eating to get fitter after you give birth. (If you do decide to try it, check with your primary care physician first — who could possibly be your BFF at this point, especially if you're breastfeeding.)

What's more, if you are feeling overpowered, always seek help. Your doctor will follow your weight at every one of your pre-birth arrangements. Discuss your interest in your goals to check whether they have proposals to assist you with downsizing — if necessary — in a way that keeps both you and child safe and healthy.

Fasting and Female Hormones

In the amazing plan of your life's health choices, checking on different avenues regarding intermittent fasting appears to be modest, correct? Tragically — for certain women, it appears as though this small decision can have huge effects on their life. Notably, the hormones directing key functions like ovulation are extraordinarily delicate to your health as a woman no matter what. The hypothalamic-pituitary-gonadal (HPG) hub — that works with the three endocrine organs — acts somewhat like an air traffic controller just like in machines.

- First, the main nerve takes out the gonadotropin-releasing hormone (GnRH)
- This advises the pituitary to take out the lutein hormone (LH) and follicular stimulating hormone (FSH)
- LH and FSH at that time follow up on the gonads such as the testicles or ovaries
- In women, this triggers the production of estrogen and progesterone — which we have to secrete a developed egg (ovulation) and to help a pregnancy

- In men, this triggers the generation of testosterone and sperm creation
- Since this chain of responses occurs on a quite certain, normal cycle in females, GnRH beats must be properly executed, or everything can get out of whack

GnRH is known to be superbly touchy to natural factors and can be lost by fasting. Indeed, even early fasting traditions (passive fasting and three-day fasts) modify hormonal levels in certain ladies. There is the possibility that missing a certain meal can begin to put us on alert, just take everything moderately and do not push your body to the limits. There are a lot of times wherein women do fine and respond well with intermittent fasting while others run into issues.

Why does intermittent fasting influence women's hormones more than men's? We're not absolutely certain. It may have something to do with a protein-like atom that neurons use to speak with one another and entirely important stuff. This protein invigorates GnRH creation in both genders, and we understand that it's remarkably sensitive to leptin, insulin, and ghrelin — hormones that manage and respond to hunger.

It is known that women have more of this hormone than guys. More hormone (kisspeptin) neurons may mean a more noteworthy effect on changes in a healthy balance. This may be one drive behind why fasting causes women's kisspeptin creation to plunge, tossing their GnRH storage.

It is important to present some studies to show the science I've been depicting here, at the same point, as I mentioned, there are none. So, all things being equal, we'll look at an ongoing report on rodents.

Intermittent fasting dietary limitation routine has an effect on proliferation in young rodents.

The point of the study comprised 10 male and 10 female common-sized rodents.

- Half the rodents ate at whatever point they needed.

- The other half ate consistently on a daily basis. In the middle of meals, their sustenance was evacuated, and they fasted.

This continued for 12 weeks, which is what could be compared to around 10 years in human life.

Before the end of the 12 weeks, the fasting female rodents had lost 19 percent of their body weight, their blood glucose levels were lower, and their ovaries had contracted. Furthermore, the test found the female rodents' hormones were higher than the males while kisspeptin creation went down in both male and female fasting rodents, in the females, LH entirely has dropped, while estradiol which is a hormone that represses GnRH in people soared to multiple times higher than the common level. The hormone that is responsible for craving, which is leptin, was several times lower than in a hungrier female rodent.

It took 10-15 days for the process to end their regenerative cycle. As such, the female rodents' hormones — both generation and hunger controlling — were absolutely altered.

What does this mean for people? It's difficult to say, but what we do think about the HPG pivot, kisspeptin, the relationship of hormones to hunger, and women's affectability to natural workings, is that credible fasting could have a comparatively emotional impact on a female human being.

You may be thinking: "So, what's the real scenario if kisspeptin drops off and I miss several periods? I'm not having children at any point in the near future." The female system and digestion are overwhelmingly interwoven. So, if you are missing periods, you can conclude that a lot of hormones have been disturbed — not only the ones that assist you with getting pregnant.

As a rule, women will, in general, consume less protein than men. Fasting women evidently will consume even less.

Eating less protein implies taking in fewer amino acids. Amino acids are expected to actuate estrogen receptors and orchestrate insulin-like protein (IGF-1) in the liver. IGF-1 triggers the uterine segregator covering to thicken and also triggers the movement of the regenerative cycle. Subsequently, low protein-diets can decrease fertility. What we expect is that estrogen isn't only for reproduction.

However, we have estrogen receptors all through our bodies to support our cerebrums, GI tract, and bones. Change the estrogen balance, and you change metabolic aptitudes such as discernment, mind-sets, absorption, recuperation, protein turnover, and skeletal system. In relation to craving and equilibrium in our health, estrogen works in a number of ways. To start with, in the brainstem, estrogen changes the peptides that signal you to feel full (cholecystokinin) or hungry (ghrelin).

In the brain, estrogen consecutively releases neurons that stop the generation of craving triggering peptides. Do something that makes your estrogen drop, and you could wind up feeling the craving to eat more foods than you would under normal conditions.

Moreover, estrogen is subsequently a key metabolic controller. The proportions of the estrogenic metabolites (estriol, estradiol, and estrone) change after some time. Prior to menopause, estradiol is a large player. After menopause, it drops, while estrone stays the same in terms of amount.

The functions of every one of these estrogens remain indistinct. Be that as it may, some speculate that a drop in estradiol may start an accumulation of the amount of fat. Why? Because fat is used to produce estradiol.

This may somehow explain why some women find it harder to lose fat after menopause. What's more, it may trigger you to think about your health — no matter if you are not focused on having children. The reason for this is that men have the ability to stroll around, do physical exercises to get ripped or push-ups to get abs. Perhaps, developmentally, you shouldn't try to get that washboard stomach in case you're female.

Low-vitality diets can decrease fertility in women. Being too lean is a conceptive hindrance. Female bodies are dazzlingly aware of health dangers and advantages. When you consider this, it bodes well.

Human females are fabulously unique in the mammalian world because early warm-blooded animals can end or delay a pregnancy basically whenever they want to. In people, the placenta breaks the maternal veins, and the baby is completely reliant on the mother when it comes to nutrients.

The child can hinder the reaction of insulin in order to store more glucose for itself. The embryo can cause the mother's veins to widen, altering the circulatory strain to get to more supplements. That child is resolved to withstand no matter what the expense to the mother. This is the reason why researchers compare it to the host-infection relationship.

When a woman gets pregnant, she can't say to the fetus to quit growing. The outcome: fertility at an inappropriate time — like, during starvation — could be lethal. No big surprise the conceptive pathway is sensitive to metabolic signals at numerous levels.

How does the body "know"? Women's hormonal balance is super sensitive to all factors. But how do our bodies "know" when there is a scarcity of food?

For a long time, experts accepted that it was a woman's muscular mass versus fat ratio that managed her regenerative system to work excellently. The thought was that if your fat stored would be burned at a particular rate (11% may be a rough estimate), hormones would fail and your period would stop.

If there isn't a lot to eat, you'll lose muscle and fat after some time. However, the circumstance is, in reality, more muddled than that. All things considered, nourishment accessibility can change rapidly. What's more, — as you most likely know, whether you've at any point attempted to get more fit — muscle versus fat regularly requires a significant stretch of time to drop, regardless of whether you're eating fewer calories.

In the interim, females who aren't predominantly lean can also quit ovulating and lose their periods. That is the reason researchers have come to speculate that overall health balance might be more essential to this method than muscle to fat ratio.

Bad overall wellbeing in women might be at fault for the hormonal domino impact we've been tackling. However, it's not just about how much food you eat.

Bad vitality balance can result from:

- Too little food consumption
- Poor nutrients
- Too much exercise
- Too much pressure
- Certain illnesses
- Too little rest and recuperation

We can even go through vitality restoration by making yourself warm. Any mix of these stressors could be enough to place you into bad health situations that can stop ovulation: preparing for a long-distance race and nursing an influenza illness, an excessive number of days straight at the gym, and eating insufficient foods.

Mental pressure can be the root cause that ruins the hormonal balance. Our bodies can't differentiate between the real hazards and something fanciful produced by our realizations and sentiments. For example, stressing over how you will get abs.

The pressure hormone cortisol hinders GnRH and stifles the ovaries' generation of estrogen and progesterone.

Moreover, progesterone is changed over to cortisol during stress; more cortisol means lower progesterone. This prompts estrogen prevalence in the HPG pivot which leads to more issues. You could be drifting at 30% fat. However, if your health balance is bad for a long-term period, especially if you're focused on weight loss alone, hormone production stops.

What to do now? In view of what we know, discontinuous skipping of meals most likely influences regenerative wellbeing if the body considers it to be a critical factor. Anything that affects your regenerative health influences your general wellness regardless of whether you plan to have children.

Moreover, feelings about intermittent fasting and results fluctuate, with some being more aggressive than others. Factors, for example, your age, your wholesome status, the timetable you fast, and different worries throughout your life—including exercise—are somehow important.

Chapter 6: Tips on Successful Intermittent Fasting

What to Eat While Practicing Intermittent Fasting?

There are no details or limitations about what type or how much food to eat while following intermittent fasting. Foods that are high in fiber, natural, entire foods that offer assortment and flavor are recommended. As it were, eat a lot of the following food sources, and you won't wind up hungry while fasting.

- **Water**

Despite the reality that you aren't eating, it's imperative to keep yourself hydrated with water for many reasons, such as for the vitality of every important organ in your body.

The amount of water that every human should consume alters. You need your urine to be a light yellow shade every time; this shows that you are hydrated. Dark yellow urine shows dehydration, which can cause cerebral pains, exhaustion, and tipsiness. Couple that with unhealthy foods, and it could be a formula for disaster. If the idea of plain water doesn't give you a boost then include a squeeze of lemon juice, some mint leaves, or cucumber cuts to your water. It'll be our little mystery.

- **Avocado**

It seems like it's irrational to eat the unhealthiest natural foods while you want to be thinner, but the monounsaturated fat in avocado is incredibly huge. A study even found that including a segment of an avocado in your lunch may keep you full for a decent length of time longer than if you didn't eat the green pearl.

- **Fish**

Every person should consume eight ounces of fish every week. In addition to the fact that it is rich in fats and protein, it also has measures of vitamin D. What's more, if there is a chance you're eating a limited amount of food throughout the day, you can consume some food supplements; however, are you getting good value for your money? Also constraining your calorie intake may upset your stomach or mind, and fish is frequently viewed as a "brain food."

- **Leafy Veggies**

Veggies like broccoli, brussels sprouts, and cauliflower are, for the most part, packed with fiber. At the point when you're eating inconsistently, it's pivotal to eat fiber-rich foods that will keep you normal and avoid blockage. It can also make you feel full, which is something you may need in case you can't eat again for 16 hours.

- **Potatoes**

Not every white food is terrible. A valid example: studies have found potatoes are not only delicious but are also comprised of healthy carbs and some vitamins. Another analysis concluded that eating potatoes as a major aspect of a good eating regimen might help with weight reduction. Apologies, but french fries and potato chips don't count.

- **Beans and Legumes**

Your likable bean stew might be your greatest friend in the intermittent fasting way of life. Beans and legumes are a good source of carbohydrates and supply energy for action. While we're not telling you to carbo-load, it certainly wouldn't hurt to include several low-calorie carbs, similar to beans and vegetables, into your eating plan. Moreover, foods such as chickpeas, dark beans, peas, and lentils have been shown to diminish excess fats, even without calorie limitation.

- **Probiotics**

You know what the little critters in your gut like the most? Consistency - because it shows that the gut wants that kind of routine but, when your gut is disturbed, you may see several aggravating reactions, similar to allergies. To balance this obnoxiousness, include probiotic-rich foods such as kefir, fermented tea, or kraut to your food consumption routine.

- **Berries**

Your favorite smoothie drink is loaded with lots of nutrients. Strawberries are an incredible source of vitamin C, 100 percent overindulgence of your everyday needs in one cup. This is not the only benefit—an ongoing study has found that people who adhered to an eating regimen that is packed in flavonoids, similar to those found in blueberries and strawberries, had lesser elevations in BMI over a 14-year span than people who didn't eat berries.

- **Eggs**

A huge egg has six grams of protein and cooks in minutes. Getting as much protein as could sensibly be expected is noteworthy for keeping full and building muscle. One study found that men who had an egg for breakfast rather than a bagel were less hungry and ate less for the extent of the day. At the end of the day, when you're probing for something to do during your fasting period, why not hard-boil some eggs?

- **Nuts**

They may be higher in calories than numerous other snacks; however, nuts contain something that most inferior food doesn't, more fat. Research suggests that polyunsaturated fat in nuts can really change the physiological markers for yearning and satiety.

What's more, let's say you're stressed over calories, don't be! A recent report found that a one-ounce serving of almonds has 20 percent fewer calories than recorded on it. Essentially, the moment you bite it doesn't wholly take apart the almond cell dividers, leaving a segment of the nut unblemished and unabsorbed during processing.

- **Whole Grains**

Being on an eating plan and eating carbs are two concepts that seem to have a place in two separate basins, however not generally! Wholegrains are wealthy in fiber and protein, so eating a little goes far in keeping you full. Additionally, another study recommends that eating whole grains rather than refined grains may really fire up your digestion. Feel free to eat your grains and venture out of your usual range of familiarity to attempt farro, bulgur, spelt, Kamut, amaranth, millet, sorghum, or freekeh.

Don'ts in Intermittent Fasting

Don't attempt to have unlimited calories during the food consumption phase. It is known that the food consumption phase gives your body the power it needs to work perfectly according to its functions. It tends to be enticing to limit calories during the food consumption phase but this can limit your improvements and result in a feeling of craving more foods. This will ruin all of your progress and waste all of your efforts.

Never practice gluttonous eating during the food consumption phase. The opposite of limiting calories is gluttonous eating. It is not recommended because you will accumulate a lot of calories and hinder you from getting the best results when fasting.

Never push your body to the limits while fasting.

Whenever you're fasting, your body is deficient in nutrients compared to your regular eating routines. While it's best to break a sweat when fasting, you should keep in mind not to overexert your body too much during those exercises.

Side Effects of Intermittent Fasting

There is a lot of proof that intermittent fasting comes with some conceivable negative effects. You shouldn't begin an intermittent fasting eating plan without working those things out with your primary care physician first.

Here are 10 warnings to keep an eye out for. If you have seen any of these reactions, it is recommended you stop intermittent fasting and speak to your primary care physician or a nutritionist before continuing.

- ## Feeling of Hungriness

We're not 100 percent sure that "hungriness" is the right term to use, but it's a very authentic sensation. This is an inclination to irritability or, generally speaking, grumpiness that happens when not having the option to eat when your body is saying to you that it's hungry.

Making your body go 16 hours without consuming anything needs some training, and a few people's bodies may not ever be glad about eating inside a limited window.

In principle, if you're consuming enough protein later in the day or night, you shouldn't feel like you're starving during your fasting period. If you feel like you're starving, that is a sign you have to make some dietary changes during your caloric intake period to restrict yourself from altering yourself into a significant twist — or it's a symptom that you're just not working well with fasting.

For some people (just like the ones who work out extensively), not eating for significant periods may not be the right fit for them, and that is simply worth considering.

- **Exhaustion**

Ever experienced yawning again and again early in the day, just to admit you never got around to having breakfast? Since not having breakfast is in general how a great many people do intermittent fasting, understanding that you're irrationally shattered each day — or making mistakes since you're swimming through your clouded brain — is a tip-off that you're not eating the proper foods during non-fasting hours or that fasting isn't going along with your way of life needs.

Always focus on what you're filling your body with. You can eat what you need on intermittent fasting, though you should at present be filling it with great sustenance that will make you feel sound and well. If you merely feel better-having breakfast most days, be mindful of your body.

- **Food Fixations**

Being on any type of prohibitive eating routine can influence your relationship with food. While some people like the amazing nature of intermittent fasting, others may end up consuming excess calories when they can eat and do not pay attention to the number of calories they're getting.

Investing too much energy into contemplating the quality or amount of your food regularly can result in a kind of dietary problem called orthorexia. It implies you focus too much on "right" or "invigorating" eating that can detrimentally affect your overall health.

That shouldn't be the primary focus of any eating practice, because you need to rely on shaping a healthy, positive relationship with foods.

- **Low Glucose**

If you're having persevering sickness, migraines, or wooziness during intermittent fasting, that is a warning that shows the eating routine may be disrupting your glucose in a bad way. People with diabetes must avoid any type of fasting diet due to this accurate explanation: intermittent fasting can make you become hypoglycemic, an unwelcome scenario for anybody with insulin or thyroid issues.

- **Male pattern baldness**

Unexpected weight reduction or the lack of real supplements, such as protein and B vitamins, can cause male pattern baldness. Since intermittent fasting doesn't want us to lose vitamins, it will surely be harder to eat a balanced diet when you're packing an entire day of eating into a few hours. If you think more hair than expected is dropping out in the shower each day, reconsider the foods that you are eating on a daily basis and talk with your physician about whether intermittent fasting is actually advantageous for you.

- **Changes in your menstrual cycle**

Here's a scenario of abrupt weight reduction (which can be a consequence of intermittent fasting): women who lose a massive amount of weight or are not getting enough calories consistently may find their menstrual cycles delayed or even stopped totally.

Girls who have an unnecessarily low body weight are inclined to an illness called amenorrhea, or the lack of a menstrual cycle. Unexpected weight reduction or being underweight can disturb your run of the hormone cycle and cause missed periods; so while you may be celebrating that intermittent fasting has helped you shed pounds, you must also be aware if it alters your menstrual cycle.

If you stop having your period and believe it's linked to the intermittent fasting methodologies you're doing, quit fasting and talk with your gynecologist to further evaluate your concern.

- **Blockage**

Any eating routine can cause an irritated stomach as you are not getting enough liquid, nutrients, protein, or fiber. It is crucial to stay replenished with liquids the entire day.

Neglecting to drink water during the fasting phase is sometimes okay, but going 16 hours every day without enough liquid is a formula for a (gastrointestinal) fiasco. So, if you've started an intermittent fasting diet and can't get your defecations to occur constantly, it's a nice way to hit stop on your preparation and first talk to a nutritionist or primary care physician about what's going on.

- **Undesirable eating routine**

Even if intermittent fasting doesn't generate a real issue like orthorexia, always be mindful of its possible effects to ensure that it will not result in critical issues. Despite not getting the right supplements, you could stop settling on bad decisions during non-fasting hours.

The primary issue is voraciously consuming food because you are so eager, you're eating 5,000 calories and going way over your daily amount.

- **Rest aggravations**

Numerous individuals have experienced a lack of sleep while doing intermittent fasting. Intermittent fasting helps control late-evening hunger, and thus, a failure to nod off if your stomach is occupied and in the process of digesting in the evening.

If you notice you can't nod off or stay unconscious after you've begun an intermittent fasting eating plan, then pause for a while and talk with an expert to ensure you're not doing something that can harm your health.

- **State of mind changes**

It would be bizarre if you did not come across any feeling of illness or hungriness during intermittent fasting in any capacity. Keep in mind that a few people feel a real health improvement or motivation once they acclimate to fasting; consider it is as a kind of constrained way of eating. Feeling committed to doing it could affect your thinking, specifically if you're away from companions or relatives because of your strict eating regimens.

However, if you're feeling down, restless, or weary about intermittent fasting, it's alright to stop and contact a certified dietitian, therapist, or nourishment mentor immediately. They can give the option to assist you with making a fasting plan that better suits your brain and body.

Is Intermittent Fasting for You?

Taking into consideration that it is still incomparable how many benefits you can get from fasting, it must always be done in moderation. This is why I would recommend a moderate methodology. If you need to attempt intermittent fasting, start with a delicate rule, and focus on how things are going.

Discontinue intermittent fasting if:

- Your menstrual cycle stops or gets sporadic
- You have issues with regards to being unconscious
- Your hair loss is getting worst
- You begin to get dry skin or breakouts
- You're noticing you don't recover from exercises as effectively as possible
- Your wounds are not healing properly because of the presence of infection in the wounds
- Your mindset starts swinging
- Your heart starts to beat in a strange manner
- Your emotions change frequently

- Your digestion is altered

- You consistently seem to feel cold

Fasting isn't for everybody. In all actuality, a few ladies ought not, in any case, try testing out intermittent fasting. Do not to attempt if:

- You're pregnant

- You have a background in eating issues such as anorexia

- You are peer pressured into trying

- You don't sleep soundly

- You're new to abstinence from food and exercise

Pregnant women have extra nutritional requirements. So, if you're beginning a family, fasting is certifiably not a smart thought. If you are under constant pressure or if you aren't recuperating properly, then your body needs sustenance, not extra pressure.

Furthermore, if you've battled with eating disorders previously, you most likely perceive that a fasting activity could lead you down a path that may create further issues for you.

It would be better for you to dig deeper into any kinds of inadequacies before you start exploring different avenues regarding fasts. Make sure you're starting from a strong dietary base first.

What to do if fasting isn't for you? How can you get fit and healthy at the same time if intermittent fasting is not a decent option for you? Become familiar with the basics of good foods. It's by far the best thing you can accomplish for your wellbeing.

- Cook and eat whole foods

- Exercise consistently

- Remain consistent in your routine

- Hire a nutritionist

Of course, intermittent fasting may be mainstream. Perhaps your family members, better half, or even your parents think it's a superb guide to wellness. However, women are not quite similar, and our bodies have various needs, you must know your body. Furthermore, do what works best for you.

Chapter 7: 7-Day Meal Plan

You can use the following meal plan below, but make sure to align it to the kind of plan you will implement, such as 16:8 or 5:2. If you are doing the 16:8 fasting plan, you can only consume the first half of the meals because you will need to set a window of 8 hours per day for food consumption while the remaining hours are devoted to fasting. You can eat the meals from breakfast up to lunch or lunch to evening or either of the two. Just make sure that it is in the eight-hour time frame.

On the other hand, if you are doing a 5:2 diet, what you should do is to omit two days from the meal plan (any days will do) as you need to eat normally for 5 days. The meals on the remaining two days should be modified by reducing your consumption so it will meet the 500 to 600 calories a day. If you are not currently fasting, you can use the meal plan as is without any modifications.

Day 1 (1316 Calories)

Breakfast: Deviled Eggs

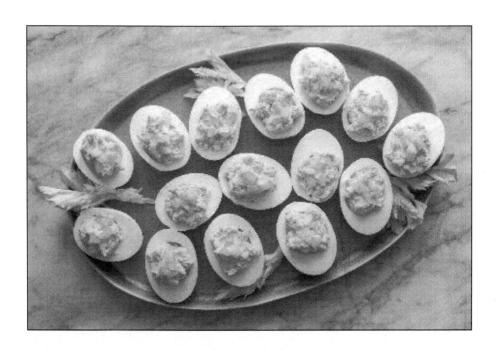

Cook Time: 20 minutes

Servings: 6

Ingredients:

- 8 oz. full-fat cream cheese, softened at room temperature

- 12 eggs

- 2 tablespoons everything bagel seasoning

- ½ teaspoon salt

- 1 grind black pepper

Instructions:

1. Add eggs to cold water, bring to a boil and cook for 10 minutes. Drain and add to cold water, let rest for 1-2 minutes. Peel the eggs.

2. Cut eggs in half lengthwise and scoop out the yolks. Add yolks to the bowl.

3. Slice cream cheese and add to the bowl with yolks. Blend well. Add in the salt and pepper and beat well.

4. Fill egg whites with the yolk mixture. Add seasoning son top. Serve.

Nutritional info (per serving): Calories 277; Total fat 22.6 g; Saturated fat 10.5 g; Protein 14.9 g; Total carbs 3.3 g; Net carbs 3.1 g; Fiber 0.2 g; Sugar 1.6 g

Lunch: Caesar Salad with Chicken

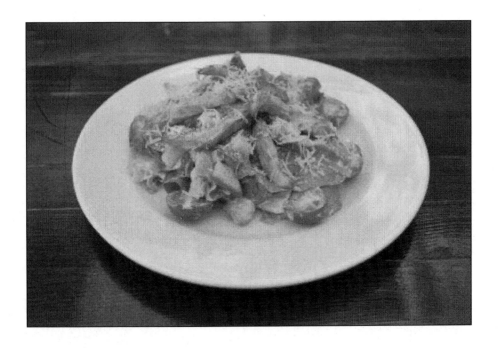

Cook Time: 15 minutes

Servings: 4

Ingredients:

- 2 chicken breasts, grilled
- 1 head Romaine lettuce, chopped
- 2 cup grape tomatoes, halved

- Parmesan cheese strips

For the Dressing:

- 3 garlic cloves, minced
- ½ lemon, juiced
- 1 ½ teaspoon Dijon mustard
- ¾ cup mayonnaise
- 1 ½ teaspoons anchovy paste
- 1 teaspoon Worcestershire sauce
- Salt and pepper, to taste

Instructions:

1. Mix all the dressing ingredients in a bowl and whisk well to combine. Cover and refrigerate the salad dressing.

2. Mix grape tomatoes, romaine lettuce and cooked chicken in a bowl. Crumble the cheese crisps into smaller pieces. Add dressing on top.

3. Toss to combine and serve.

Nutritional info (per serving): Calories 400; Total fat 25 g; Saturated fat 12 g; Protein 33 g; Total carbs 9 g; Net carbs 5 g; Fiber 4 g; Sugar 4 g

Snack: Coconut Chocolate Chip Cookies

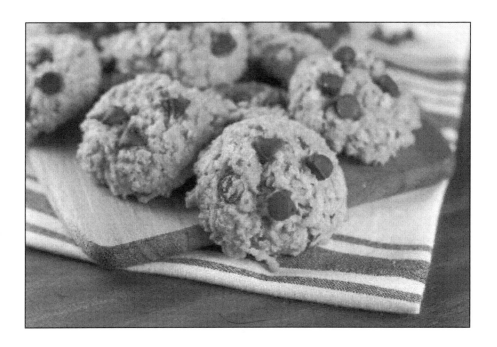

Cook Time: 30 minutes

Servings: 6

Ingredients:

- ¾ cup coconut, shredded
- 1 ¼ cups almond flour
- 1 teaspoon baking powder

- ½ cup butter (softened)

- ½ cup Swerve sweetener

- ½ teaspoon vanilla extract

- 1 egg

- ½ cup chocolate chips, sugar-free

- ½ teaspoon salt

Instructions:

1. Preheat the oven to 325°F and line a baking sheet with parchment paper.

2. Mix coconut, almond flour, baking powder, and salt in a bowl.

3. Mix butter with sweetener in a separate bowl. Beat in egg and vanilla. Stir to combine. Add this mixture to the flour mixture and beat in well. Add in the chocolate chips.

4. Shape the dough into 1 ½-inch balls. Place on the baking sheet 2 inches apart. Press each ball to ¼-inch thick.

5. Bake for 15 minutes. Remove from the oven and cool completely. Serve.

Nutritional info (per serving): Calories 268; Total fat 17.4 g; Saturated fat 10.3 g; Protein 12 g; Total carbs 13 g; Net carbs 12 g; Fiber 1 g; Sugar 10 g

Dinner: Balsamic Chicken with Roasted Vegetables

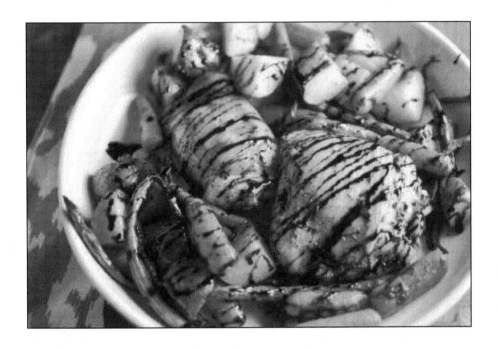

Cook Time: 30 minutes

Servings: 4

Ingredients:

- 10 asparaguses, ends trimmed and cut in half
- 8 boneless, skinless chicken thighs, fat trimmed
- 2 bell peppers, sliced into strips

- ½ cup carrots, sliced into half long and cut into 3-inch pieces
- 1 red onion, chopped into large chunks
- ¼ cup + 1 tablespoon balsamic vinegar
- 5 oz. mushrooms, sliced
- 2 tablespoons olive oil
- ½ tablespoon dried oregano
- 2 sage leaves, chopped
- 2 garlic cloves, smashed and chopped
- ½ teaspoon sugar
- 1 ½ tablespoons rosemary
- 1 teaspoon salt
- Black pepper, to taste
- Cooking spray

Instructions:

1. Preheat the oven to 425°F.
2. Season chicken with salt and pepper and spray 2 large baking sheets with cooking spray.

3. Mix all the ingredients in a bowl and mix well. Place everything on the prepared baking sheet and spread in a single layer.

4. Bake for 25 minutes. Serve.

Nutritional info (per serving): Calories 450; Total fat 17 g; Saturated fat 3 g; Protein 48 g; Total carbs 15 g; Net carbs 4 g; Fiber 11 g; Sugar 2 g

Day 2 (1358 Calories)

Breakfast: Cream Cheese Pancakes

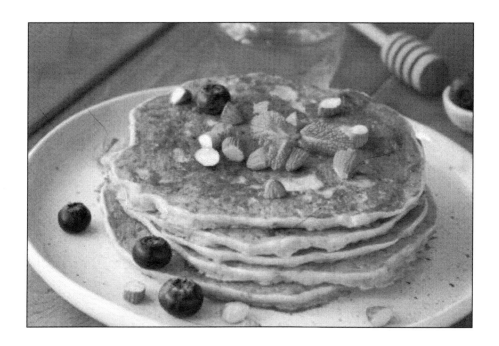

Cook Time: 15 minutes

Servings: 2

Ingredients:

- 2 eggs
- 4 oz. cream cheese

- ½ teaspoon baking powder
- ¼ cup almond flour
- ¼ teaspoon fine salt
- Cooking spray

Instructions:

1. Mix eggs, flour, cream cheese, baking powder, and salt in a blender and blend until smooth.

2. Heat a frying pan over medium heat and grease with cooking spray. Add 3 tablespoons batter. Cook for 3 minutes. Flip and cook for 2 more minutes. Transfer to a plate.

3. Repeat with the remaining batter. Serve.

Nutritional info (per serving): Calories 329; Total fat 30.2 g; Saturated fat 16.7 g; Protein 10.1 g; Total carbs 5.4 g; Net carbs 4.2 g; Fiber 1.3 g; Sugar 2.9 g

Lunch: Thai Beef Salad

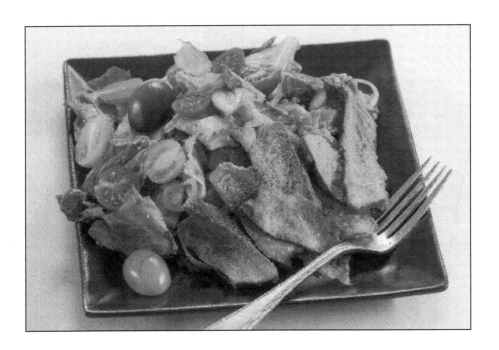

Cook Time: 15 minutes

Servings: 4

Ingredients:

- 1 ½ lb. flank steak

- 1 tablespoon olive oil

- 1 teaspoon sea salt

- 1 cup cucumbers, chopped
- 1 head lettuce, chopped
- 1 cup grape tomatoes, halved
- ¼ cup basil, cut into ribbons
- ¼ cup cilantro, chopped
- ¼ cup red onion, sliced
- ¼ cup olive oil
- ¼ cup coconut aminos
- 1 tablespoon fish sauce
- 2 tablespoon lime juice
- 1 tablespoon Thai red curry paste

Instructions:

1. Mix oil, coconut aminos, fish sauce, lime juice, and curry paste in a bowl and whisk to combine.
2. Season steak with salt on all sides. Put steak slices in a single layer into a glass baking dish. Add half of the marinade over the steak.

3. Cover meat with plastic wrap and refrigerate for 8 hours. Cover the reserved dressing and refrigerate.

4. Mix lettuce, cucumbers, grape tomatoes, cilantro, red onion, and basil in a bowl. Cook beef in a hot pan until brown on all sides. Let beef rest for 5 minutes. Slice against the grain.

5. Serve salad with beef and dressing.

Nutritional info (per serving): Calories 426; Total fat 26 g; Saturated fat 14.2 g; Protein 38 g; Total carbs 8 g; Net carbs 7 g; Fiber 1 g; Sugar 2 g

Snack: Buffalo Chicken Sausage Balls

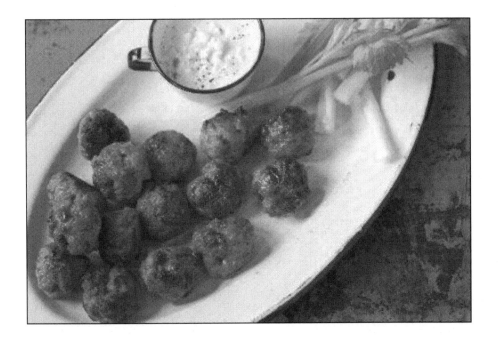

Cook Time: 40 minutes

Servings: 12 balls

Ingredients:

- 3 tablespoons coconut flour

- 24 oz. bulk chicken sausage

- 1 cup cheddar cheese, shredded

- 1 cup almond flour
- ½ cup Buffalo wing sauce
- ½ teaspoon cayenne
- 1 teaspoon salt
- ½ teaspoon pepper
- 2 garlic cloves, minced
- 1 teaspoon dried dill
- 1/3 cup mayonnaise
- 1/3 cup almond milk, unsweetened
- ½ teaspoon dried parsley
- ¼ cup bleu cheese, crumbled
- ½ teaspoon salt
- ½ teaspoon pepper

Instructions:

1. Preheat the oven to 350°F and line 2 baking sheets with parchment paper.

2. Mix cheddar cheese, sausage, almond flour, coconut flour, buffalo sauce, cayenne, salt, and pepper in a bowl and mix well until combined.

3. Roll the mixture into 1-inch balls and place on the baking sheets 1 inch apart. Bake for 25 minutes.

4. Mix mayo, almond milk, garlic, parsley, dill, salt, and pepper in a bowl. Mix well and add bleu cheese in. Mix well.

5. Serve balls with the sauce.

Nutritional info (per serving): Calories 255; Total fat 19.3 g; Saturated fat 4.7 g; Protein 15.3 g; Total carbs 4.2 g; Net carbs 2.5 g; Fiber 1.7 g; Sugar 5 g

Dinner: Low Carb Chili

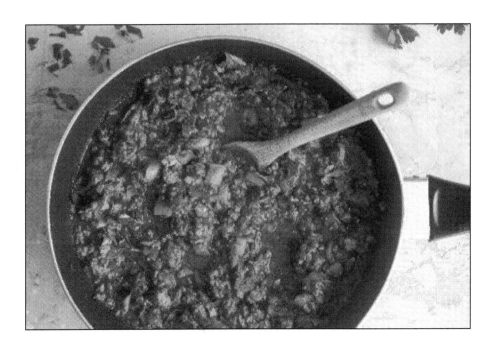

Cook Time: 40 minutes

Servings: 6

Ingredients:

- 1 bell pepper, chopped

- 1 ¼ lb. ground beef

- 8 oz. tomato paste

- 1 ½ tomato, chopped

- 2 celery sticks, chopped

- ½ cup onion, chopped

- 1 ½ teaspoons cumin

- ¾ cup of water

- 1 ½ teaspoon chili powder

- 1 ½ teaspoons salt

- ½ teaspoon pepper

Instructions:

1. Cook the meat in a frying pan until brown. Drain the excess fat and season meat with salt.

2. Add peppers and onions to the pan and cook for 2 minutes. Mix onions, cooked meat, peppers, tomatoes, water, celery, and tomato paste in a pot.

3. Add the spices to the pot. Bring to a boil and reduce the heat to low-medium. Cook for 2 hours while stirring every 30 minutes. Serve.

Nutritional info (per serving): Calories 348; Total fat 28.8 g; Saturated fat 8.5 g; Protein 14.9 g; Total carbs 7.2 g; Net carbs 5.2 g; Fiber 2 g; Sugar 3.3 g

Day 3 (1471 Calories)

Breakfast: Oat-Free Porridge

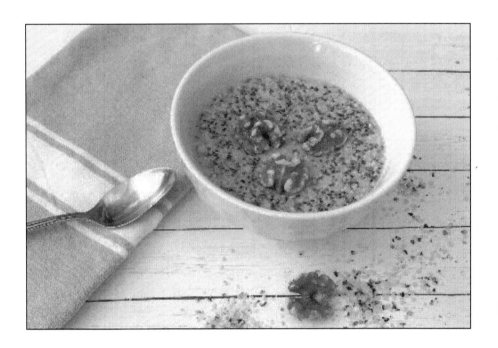

Cook Time: 5 minutes

Servings: 1

Ingredients:

- 2 tablespoons unsweetened coconut, shredded
- ½ cup of water

- 2 tablespoons hemp hearts

- 2 tablespoons almond flour

- 1 tablespoon chia seeds

- 1 tablespoon golden flaxseed meal

- ¼ teaspoon granulated stevia

- ½ teaspoon pure vanilla extract

- 1 pinch salt

Instructions:

1. Add all ingredients except vanilla to a saucepan.

2. Cook over low heat for 5 minutes, stirring constantly. Add in the vanilla. Serve.

Nutritional info (per serving): Calories 453; Total fat 36 g; Saturated fat 10 g; Protein 18 g; Total carbs 15 g; Net carbs 5 g; Fiber 10 g; Sugar 1 g

Lunch: Caprese Zucchini Noodle Pasta Salad

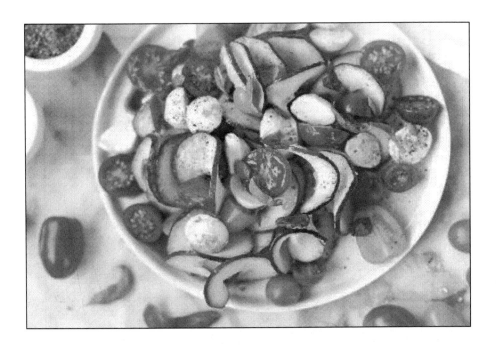

Cook Time: 15 minutes

Servings: 8 cups

Ingredients:

- 8 oz. mozzarella pearls
- 1 oz. basil, chopped

- 4 zucchinis, spiralized
- 4 oz. cherry tomatoes, sliced in half
- 3 tablespoon red wine vinegar
- ¼ cup extra virgin olive oil
- 1 tablespoon lemon juice
- ¼ teaspoon garlic powder
- ½ teaspoon salt
- ¼ teaspoon pepper

Instructions:

1. Whisk red wine, oil, lemon juice, garlic powder, salt, and pepper in a bowl.
2. Add the remaining ingredients to a bowl and add dressing on top. Toss well to combine. Serve.

Nutritional info (per serving): Calories 186; Total fat 13 g; Saturated fat 4 g; Protein 7 g; Total carbs 4 g; Net carbs 3 g; Fiber 1 g; Sugar 3 g

Snack: Bacon and Guacamole Fat Bombs

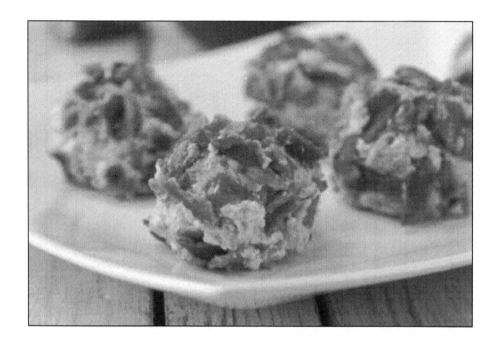

Cook Time: 45 minutes

Servings: 6

Ingredients:

- ¼ cup butter (softened)

- ½ avocado

- 2 garlic cloves, crushed

- ½ small white onion, diced

- 1 small chili pepper, finely chopped

- 1 tablespoon lime juice

- 2 tablespoons cilantro, chopped

- 4 slices bacon

- ¼ teaspoon sea salt

- Black pepper

Instructions:

1. Preheat the oven to 375°F and line a baking tray with baking paper. Place the bacon strips on the baking tray.

2. Bake for 15 minutes. Remove the tray from the oven and let cool. Crumble the bacon.

3. Cut avocado in half, remove the pit and peel it. Add butter, avocado, chili pepper, cilantro, crushed garlic, and lime juice to a bowl. Season with salt and pepper. Mash with a fork until combined.

4. Add onion and mix. Add bacon grease from the baking tray and mix well. Cover with foil and refrigerate for 30 minutes.

5. Shape the guacamole mixture into 6 balls. Roll each ball into the bacon pieces and place on a tray. Serve.

Nutritional info (per serving): Calories 156; Total fat 15.2 g; Saturated fat 6.8 g; Protein 3.4 g; Total carbs 2.7 g; Net carbs 1.4 g; Fiber 1.3 g; Sugar 0.5 g

Dinner: Cheesy Tuna Pesto Pasta

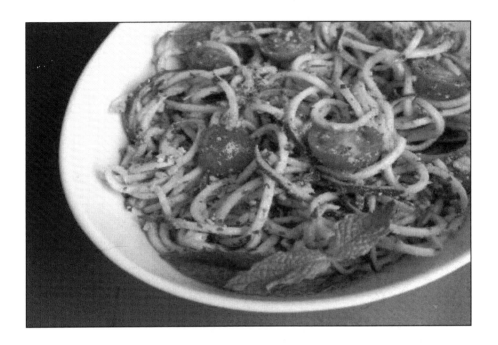

Cook Time: 25 minutes

Servings: 4

Ingredients:

- 4 cups zucchini noodles, spiralized, cooked
- 1 cup cheddar, grated
- 1 cup yellowfin tuna in olive oil

- 7 oz. basil pesto

- 1 ½ cup punnet cherry tomato, halved

Instructions:

1. Mix pesto and tuna with oil in a bowl. Mash well. Add in 1/3 of the cheese and add all the tomatoes.

2. Add noodles to the bowl, toss well to coat. Transfer the mixture to a baking dish and add the remaining cheese on top.

3. Broil the dish for 4 minutes. Serve.

Nutritional info (per serving): Calories 696; Total fat 27 g; Saturated fat 11 g; Protein 40 g; Total carbs 14 g; Net carbs 10 g; Fiber 4 g; Sugar 5 g

Day 4 (1521 Calories)

Breakfast: Keto Breakfast Bowl

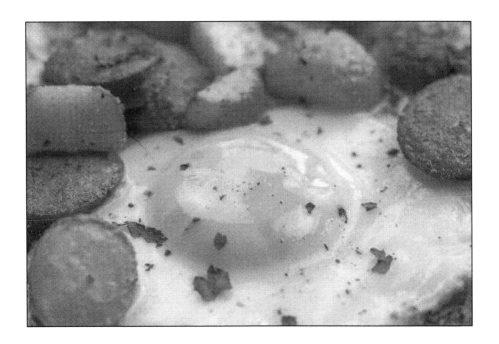

Cook Time: 30 minutes

Servings: 1

Ingredients:

- 1 egg
- ¼ cup cheddar cheese, shredded

- 2 cups radishes

- 3 ½ oz. ground sausage

- ¼ teaspoon pink Himalayan salt

- ¼ teaspoon black pepper

Instructions:

1. Cook sausage in a pan over medium high heat until done. Remove sausage the pan and set aside.

2. Cut radishes into small pieces and add to the pan. Season well. Cook radishes for 12 minutes.

3. Fry the egg the way you want and set aside. Layer the radishes with sausage on a plate, top with egg and cheese. Serve.

Nutritional info (per serving): Calories 617; Total fat 49 g; Saturated fat 11.1 g; Protein 32 g; Total carbs 7 g; Net carbs 4 g; Fiber 3 g; Sugar 5 g

Lunch: Kale and Brussels Sprout Salad

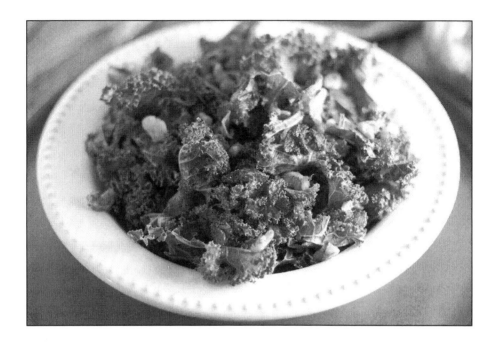

Cook Time: 15 minutes

Servings: 8

Ingredients:

- ½ lb. Brussels sprouts, outer leaves and stems removed
- ½ bunch curly kale
- 6 slices cooked bacon

- ½ cup dried cranberries
- ½ cup walnuts
- 2 tablespoons lemon juice
- 1/3 cup olive oil
- ½ teaspoon garlic powder
- 1 tablespoon Dijon mustard
- ¼ teaspoon sea salt
- ¼ teaspoon black pepper

Instructions:

1. Add Brussels sprouts to a blender and blend well until chopped.
2. Add kale leaves to it and pulse until shredded.
3. Whisk mustard, olive oil, lemon juice, garlic powder, salt, and pepper in a bowl until well mixed.
4. Add kale and Brussels sprouts and stir to combine. Add the cooked bacon, walnuts, and cranberries in it. Toss well. Serve.

Nutritional info (per serving): Calories 192; Total fat 17 g; Saturated fat 1.6 g; Protein 6 g; Total carbs 6 g; Net carbs 4 g; Fiber 2 g; Sugar 3 g

Snack: Cheddar Jalapeno Meatballs

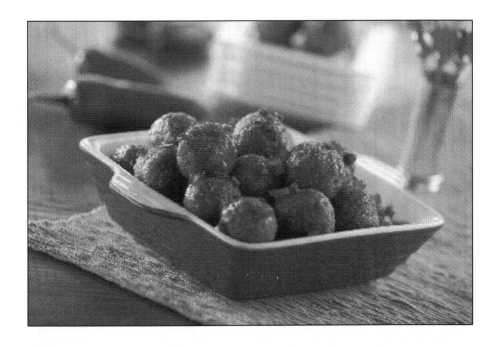

Cook Time: 45 minutes

Servings: 8

Ingredients:

- 1 ½ lb. ground beef
- 1 large jalapeno, sliced
- 6 oz. sharp cheddar, grated

- ½ cup pork rind crumbs

- 1 egg

- 1 teaspoon chili powder

- 2 tablespoons cilantro, chopped

- 1 teaspoon garlic powder

- ½ teaspoon cumin

- 1 teaspoon salt

- ½ teaspoon pepper

Instructions:

1. Preheat the oven to 375°F and line a rimmed baking sheet with parchment paper.

2. Mix all ingredients in a blender. Blend on high until well combined. Roll the dough into 1 ½-inch balls and add to the baking sheet 1 inch apart.

3. Bake for 20 minutes. Serve.

Nutritional info (per serving): Calories 368; Total fat 24 g; Saturated fat 9.7 g; Protein 33.4 g; Total carbs 1.1 g; Net carbs 0.8 g; Fiber 0.3 g; Sugar 1 g

Dinner: Keto Meatloaf

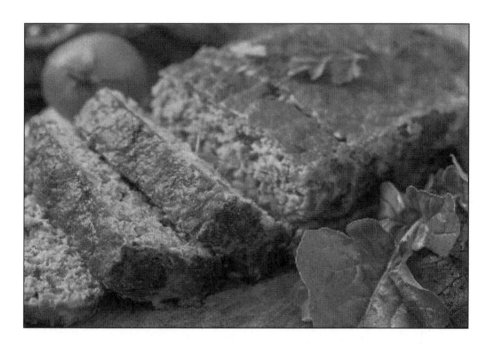

Cook Time: 1 hour

Servings: 6

Ingredients:

- 2 eggs
- 2 lbs. 85% lean grass-fed ground beef
- ¼ cup nutritional yeast

- 1 tablespoon lemon zest

- 2 tablespoons avocado oil

- ¼ cup parsley, chopped

- 4 garlic cloves

- ¼ cup oregano, chopped

- ½ tablespoon pink Himalayan salt

- 1 teaspoon black pepper

Instructions:

1. Preheat the oven to 400°F. Mix beef, yeast, salt, and pepper in a bowl.

2. Mix eggs, oil, garlic, and herbs in a blender and blend until everything is mixed well. Add this mixture to the beef and mix well.

3. Add the beef mixture to a small loaf pan. Arrange the pan on the middle rack and bake for 1 hour. Remove the pan from the oven. Let cool for 10 minutes. Serve.

Nutritional info (per serving): Calories 344; Total fat 29 g; Saturated fat 13.4 g; Protein 33 g; Total carbs 4 g; Net carbs 2 g; Fiber 2 g; Sugar 1 g

Day 5 (1371 Calories)

Breakfast: Sausage and Peppers No Egg Breakfast Bake

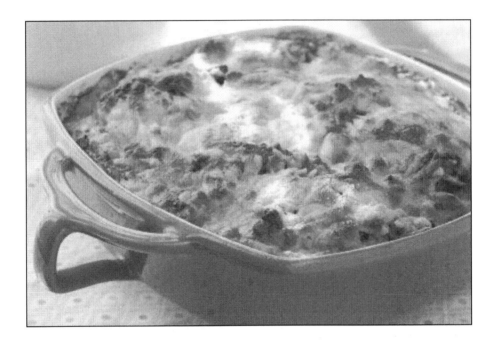

Cook Time: 50 minutes

Servings: 4

Ingredients:

- 1 ½ teaspoon olive oil

- 1 green bell pepper, chopped

- 1 red bell pepper, chopped

- ½ cup mozzarella cheese, grated

- 10 oz. sausage

- Salt, black pepper, to taste

Instructions:

1. Preheat the oven to 450°F and grease a medium-sized dish with cooking spray.

2. Add peppers to the baking dish and toss with 1 teaspoon olive oil and add salt and black pepper on top. Bake for 20 minutes.

3. Heat remaining olive oil on a pan and add the sausages. Cook over medium-high heat for 12 minutes.

4. Cut sausages into pieces. Add the sausages to the baking pan with the peppers. Bake for 5 more minutes.

5. Remove the dish from the oven, turn the oven to broil. Add the mozzarella over the peppers and sausages. Broil for 2 minutes. Serve.

Nutritional info (per serving): Calories 246; Total fat 13 g; Saturated fat 5 g; Protein 26 g; Total carbs 5 g; Net carbs 4 g; Fiber 1 g; Sugar 2 g

Lunch: Curried Cabbage Coconut Salad

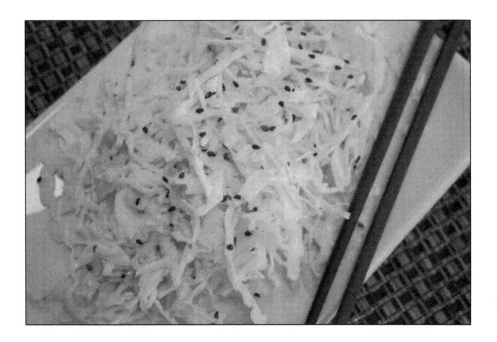

Cook Time: 5 minutes

Servings: 4

Ingredients:

- ¼ cup of coconut oil

- ½ head white cabbage, shredded

- 1 lemon juice

- 1/3 cup dried coconut, unsweetened
- ¼ cup tamari sauce (like Soy Sauce but less Salty, Thickerd Then Soy Sauce - Can also Substitute Fish Saucer Coconut Aminos
- ½ teaspoon ginger, dried
- 3 teaspoons sesame seeds
- ½ teaspoon curry powder
- ½ teaspoon cumin

Instructions:

1. Add all the ingredients to a bowl and toss well.

2. Cover and refrigerate for 1 hour. Serve.

Nutritional info (per serving): Calories 309; Total fat 5 g; Saturated fat 8 g; Protein 12 g; Total carbs 12 g; Net carbs 6 g; Fiber 6 g; Sugar 3 g

Snack: Cheesy Party Crackers

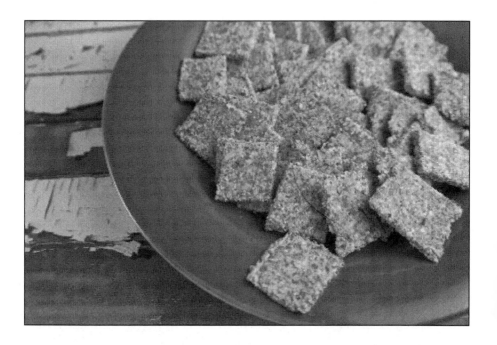

Cook Time: 45 minutes

Servings: 8

Ingredients:

- ½ cup flax meal
- 1 cup almond flour
- 2 tablespoons whole psyllium husks

- 1 cup of water

- 1 cup Parmesan cheese, grated

- 1 teaspoon salt

- ¼ teaspoon black pepper

Instructions:

1. Mix flax meal, almond flour, psyllium, salt, and pepper in a bowl. Add the cheese to it and mix well. Add water and mix well. Let rest for 15 minutes.

2. Preheat the oven to 320°F and divide the dough into 2 parts.

3. Place half of the dough on a parchment paper. Place another piece of parchment paper on top and roll the dough out until thin.

4. Cut the dough into 16 equal pieces. Repeat the process with the remaining dough.

5. Bake for 45 minutes. Serve.

Nutritional info (per serving): Calories 169; Total fat 13.4 g; Saturated fat 2.7 g; Protein 8.4 g; Total carbs 6.3 g; Net carbs 1.7 g; Fiber 4.5 g; Sugar 0.8 g

Dinner: Crispy Salmon with Pesto Cauliflower Rice

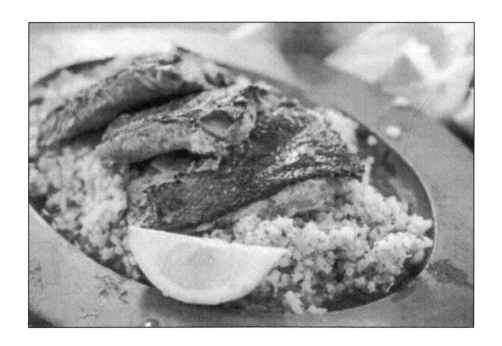

Cook Time: 40 minutes

Servings: 3

Ingredients:

- 1 tablespoon olive oil
- 3 salmon fillets

- 1 tablespoon coconut aminos
- 1 teaspoon fish sauce
- 1 tablespoon butter
- 3 garlic cloves
- 1 cup basil leaves, chopped
- ¼ cup hemp hearts
- ½ cup olive oil
- 1 lemon juice
- ½ teaspoon pink salt
- 3 cups riced cauliflower, frozen
- 1 scoop MCT Powder
- Pinch salt

Instructions:

1. Add fish sauce, coconut aminos, and olive oil to a baking dish. Pat the salmon fillets dry and add place into the dish skin side down. Add a pinch of salt. Let rest for 20 minutes.

2. Heat an iron skillet on medium heat.

3. Peel and dice the garlic and add it to a blender. Add hemp hearts, basil, lemon juice, olive oil, MCT powder, and salt. Pulse well to combine.

4. Heat cauliflower rice in a skillet. Add pesto and pink salt. Mix well to combine. Lower the heat and keep it warm.

5. Add butter to the iron skillet placed over medium heat. Add salmon skin side down. Cook for 5 minutes. Flip the salmon and add the remaining marinade from the plate. Sear for 2 minutes.

6. Remove from heat and serve on top of rice. Enjoy!

Nutritional info (per serving): Calories 647; Total fat 51 g; Saturated fat 10.8 g; Protein 33.8 g; Total carbs 8 g; Net carbs 5 g; Fiber 3 g; Sugar 3 g

Day 6 (1237 Calories)

Breakfast: Bacon and Egg Breakfast Muffins

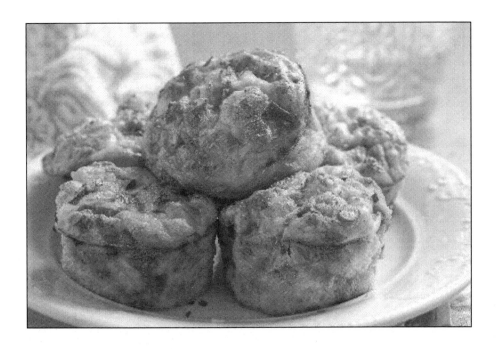

Cooking time: 25 minutes

Servings: 12

Ingredients:

- 8 eggs

- 8 bacon slices

- 2/3 cup green onion, chopped

- Cooking spray

Instructions:

1. Coat the muffin tin with nonstick cooking spray and preheat the oven to 350°F.

2. Add bacon to a large pan and cook over medium heat until crisp. Transfer to a plate lined with paper towels. Let cool and then chop into small pieces.

3. Add eggs to a bowl and whisk well. Then add green onions and cooked bacon. Mix until everything is well-combined.

4. Add the mixture to the muffin tin. Bake for about 20-25 minutes, until edges are golden brown.

5. Let the muffins cool and enjoy bacon and egg breakfast muffins.

Nutritional info (per serving): Calories 158; Total fat 13.3 g; Saturated fat 1.7 g; Protein 8 g; Total carbs 1 g; Net carbs 1 g; Fiber 0 g; Sugar 1 g

Lunch: Grilled Chicken Salad

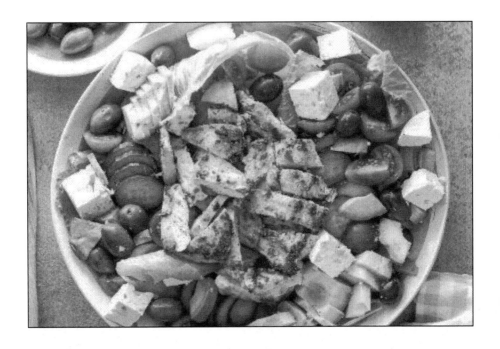

Cooking time: 20 minutes

Servings: 2

Ingredients:

- ½ lb. chicken thigh, grilled and sliced

- 1 teaspoon fresh thyme

- 4 cups romaine lettuce, chopped

- 2 garlic cloves, crushed

- 1/4 cup cherry tomatoes, chopped

- 3 tablespoons extra virgin olive oil

- ½ cucumber, thinly sliced

- 2 tablespoons red wine vinegar

- ½ avocado, sliced

- 1 oz. olives, pitted and sliced

- 1 oz. Feta cheese, crumbled

- Salt, pepper, to taste

Instructions:

1. Season chicken with a teaspoon of thyme, crushed garlic, pepper, and salt.

2. Preheat oil in a pan over medium heat. Cook chicken until golden brown.

3. Mix olives, sliced cucumber, chopped lettuce, sliced avocado, and ¼ cup tomatoes in a large bowl.

4. Add chicken to the salad. Sprinkle with crumbled cheese.

5. Drizzle with olive oil and vinegar. Enjoy!

Nutritional info (per serving): Calories 617; Total fat 52 g; Saturated fat 4 g; Protein 30 g; Total carbs 11 g; Net carbs 7 g; Fiber 4 g; Sugar 2.5 g

Snack: Keto Almond Bark

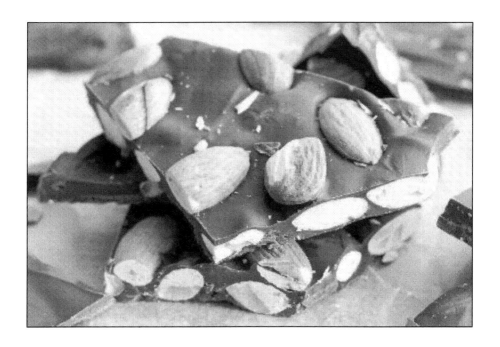

Cooking time: 15 minutes

Servings: 20

Ingredients:

- 4 oz. cocoa butter
- ½ cup Swerve sweetener
- ½ teaspoon vanilla extract

- 2 tablespoons water

- ¾ cup cocoa powder

- 1 tablespoon butter

- ½ cup powdered Swerve sweetener

- 1 ½ cups roasted almonds, unsalted

- 2 ½ oz. unsweetened chocolate, chopped

- ¼ teaspoon sea salt

Instructions:

1. Add 2 tablespoons water and ½ cup Swerve sweetener to a saucepan. Bring the mixture to a light boil, stirring occasionally. Cook for about 8 to 9 minutes until the mixture darkens.

2. Turn the heat off and whisk in 1 tablespoon butter. Add 1 ½ cups roasted almonds and toss well until coated. Then stir in 2 pinches of salt.

3. Spread almonds onto a parchment-lined baking sheet. Add 4 oz. cocoa butter and 2 ½ oz. unsweetened chocolate to a large saucepan. Melt over medium heat and stir until smooth.

4. Stir in ¾ cup cocoa powder and ½ cup powdered Swerve sweetener until smooth. Turn the heat off and stir in ½ teaspoon vanilla extract.

5. Reserve 4 tablespoons of almonds and keep them aside. Add leftover almonds to the chocolate mixture and stir well.

6. Spread chocolate-almond mixture out onto the same baking sheet. Top with reserved ¼ cups of almonds and sprinkle with salt.

7. Chill for about 3 hours and then break into chunks. Serve right away!

Nutritional info (per serving): Calories 144; Total fat 14 g; Saturated fat 1.3 g; Protein 13 g; Total carbs 5 g; Net carbs 2 g; Fiber 3 g; Sugar 10 g

Dinner: Chicken Parmesan

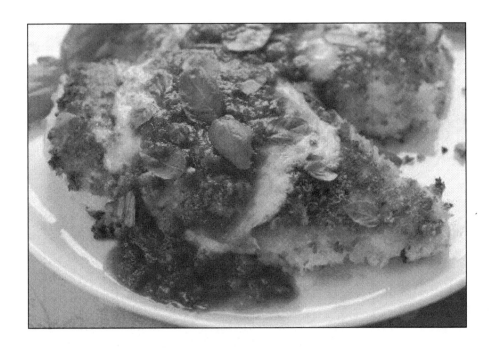

Cooking time: 19 minutes

Servings: 8

Ingredients:

- 2 lbs. boneless skinless chicken breast

- 4 oz. fresh mozzarella

- 1/3 cup sugar-free marinara

- 1 cup almond flour

- 1 cup parmesan cheese, grated

- 2 eggs

- 1 teaspoon Italian seasoning

- ½ teaspoon black pepper

- ½ teaspoon sea salt

Instructions:

1. Add chicken to a plastic bag and pound until about ½-inch thick.

2. Add 1 teaspoon Italian seasoning, a cup of parmesan cheese, ½ teaspoon sea salt, a cup of almond, and ½ teaspoon pepper. Mix well.

3. Add eggs to a separate bowl and whisk well. Pat dry the chicken with paper towels.

4. Dip chicken into the egg mixture and then coat with almond flour mixture. Brush with oil or coat with cooking spray.

5. Preheat the oven to 425°F. Place chicken on a baking sheet lined with parchment paper. Cook for about 11-12 minutes.

6. Then flip the chicken, spray with cooking spray and cook for 5 minutes more.

7. Sprinkle each piece with mozzarella and drizzle with pasta sauce. Transfer back to the oven and cook for a few minutes until cheese is melted.

Nutritional info (per serving): Calories 318; Total fat 17 g; Saturated fat 5 g; Protein 36 g; Total carbs 4 g; Net carbs 3 g; Fiber 1 g; Sugar 1 g

Day 7 (1258 Calories)

Breakfast: Chocolate Mint Avocado Smoothie

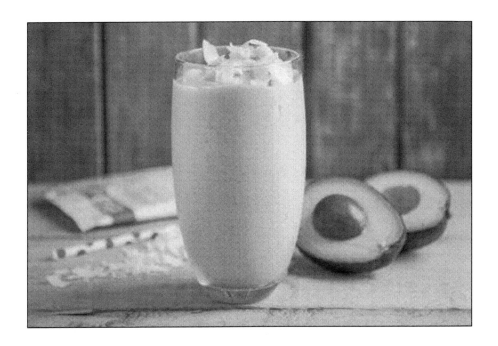

Cooking time: 5 minutes

Servings: 1

Ingredients:

- 2 scoops chocolate collagen protein

- 2 tablespoons coconut, shredded

- ½ cup of coconut milk

- 1 tablespoon cacao butter, crushed

- 1 cup of water

- 4 mint leaves

- ½ cup ice

- ½ a frozen avocado

Instructions:

1. Add all the ingredients *except* for shredded coconut and collagen protein to a blender.

2. Blend on high for about 45 seconds. Then add collagen protein to a blender and blend for 5 seconds more.

3. Top chocolate mint avocado smoothie with coconut flakes. Enjoy!

Nutritional info (per serving): Calories 552; Total fat 44 g; Saturated fat 25 g; Protein 26 g; Total carbs 10 g; Net carbs 1 g; Fiber 9 g; Sugar 2 g

Lunch: Italian Salad

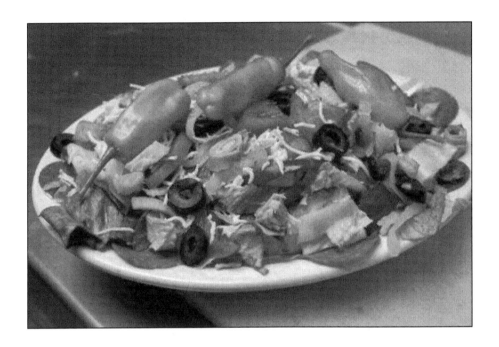

Cooking time: 15 minutes

Servings: 4

Ingredients:

- 1 cup mixed Italian olives, pitted

- 6 oz. deli ham, diced

- 6 cups Romaine lettuce, shredded

- ¼ cup pickled banana peppers, sliced

- 2 medium Roma tomatoes, diced

- ¼ red onion, sliced

  For the Vinaigrette:

- 1 tablespoon red wine vinegar

- 1 tablespoon Italian seasoning

- ½ cup olive oil

- A pinch of sea salt

- Black pepper, to taste

Instructions:

1. Add all vinaigrette ingredients to a bowl and whisk well to combine.

2. Arrange all the salad ingredients in a large bowl and top with the dressing. Toss well to combine. Enjoy!

Nutritional info (per serving): Calories 289; Total fat 24 g; Saturated fat 7 g; Protein 11 g; Total carbs 7 g; Net carbs 4 g; Fiber 3 g; Sugar 3 g

Snack: Brussels Sprouts Chips

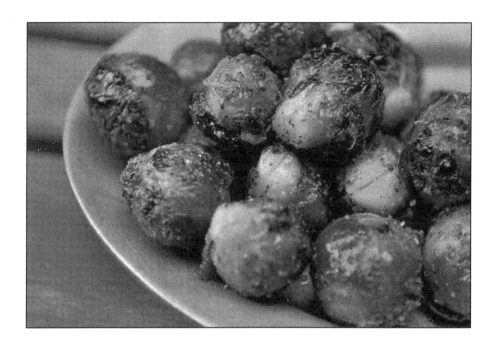

Cooking time: 15-20 minutes

Servings: 4

Ingredients:

- 1 lb. Brussels sprouts washed and dried, ends trimmed

- 1 teaspoon salt

- 2 tablespoons extra virgin olive oil

- Smoked paprika, for serving

Instructions:

1. Preheat the oven to 400°F

2. Peel the outer leaves of the Brussels sprouts and discard them. Add the sprouts to a bowl.

3. Drizzle with oil and toss well to coat in oil. Season with salt. Spread on a baking sheet evenly in one layer.

4. Bake for about 12-15 minutes. Take them out from the oven and let them cool.

5. Sprinkle with more salt if you want. Serve topped with smoked paprika.

Nutritional info (per serving): Calories 104; Total fat 7 g; Saturated fat 1.4 g; Protein 3 g; Total carbs 9 g; Net carbs 5 g; Fiber 4 g; Sugar 1 g

Dinner: Mushroom Bacon Skillet

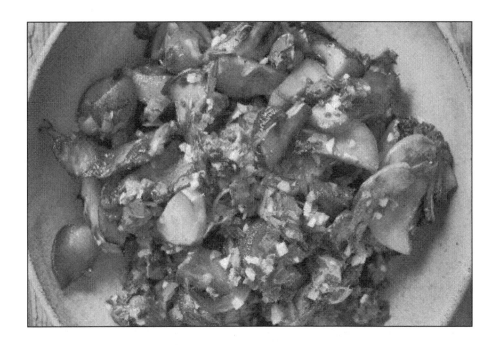

Cooking time: 10 minutes

Servings: 1

Ingredients:

- ½ teaspoon salt

- 1 tablespoon garlic, minced

- 4 slices pastured pork bacon, cut into ½-inch pieces

- 2 sprigs thyme, leaves only

- 2 cups mushrooms, halved

Instructions:

1. Preheat a skillet over medium heat. Add bacon and cook until crispy. Remove from the pan.

2. Add sliced mushrooms. Sauté until soften, stirring often.

3. Add garlic, thyme, and salt. Cook for 5 minutes more, stirring often.

4. When mushrooms become golden, turn the heat off.

5. Garnish mushroom bacon with greens and enjoy!

Nutritional info (per serving): Calories 313; Total fat 8.5 g; Saturated fat 3.8 g; Protein 13.6 g; Total carbs 8.4 g; Net carbs 0.3 g; Fiber 8.1 g; Sugar 2.2 g

Conclusion

We have finished tackling this wonderful topic about intermittent fasting. I hope you have learned a lot and found useful information. The next thing you must do now is to apply what you have learned and utilize it to your own advantage. Once you have mastered the act of intermittent fasting, you can add some twists to it, making your progress much faster and optimized. Do not hesitate to scan through the material from time to time in case you have forgotten something in order to refresh your knowledge as necessary.

Conversion Tables

VOLUME EQUIVALENTS (LIQUID)

US STANDARD	US STANDARD (OUNCES)	METRIC (APPROXIMATE)
2 tablespoons	1 fl. oz.	30 mL
¼ cup	2 fl. oz.	60 mL
½ cup	4 fl. oz.	120 mL
1 cup	8 fl. oz.	240 mL
1½ cups	12 fl. oz.	355 mL
2 cups or 1 pint	16 fl. oz.	475 mL
4 cups or 1 quart	32 fl. oz.	1 L
1 gallon	128 fl. oz.	4 L

VOLUME EQUIVALENTS (DRY)

US STANDARD	METRIC (APPROXIMATE)
⅛ teaspoon	0.5 mL
¼ teaspoon	1 mL
½ teaspoon	2 mL
¾ teaspoon	4 mL
1 teaspoon	5 mL
1 tablespoon	15 mL
¼ cup	59 mL
⅓ cup	79 mL
½ cup	118 mL
⅔ cup	156 mL
¾ cup	177 mL
1 cup	235 mL
2 cups or 1 pint	475 mL
3 cups	700 mL
4 cups or 1 quart	1 L

TEMPERATURES

FAHRENHEIT (F)	CELSIUS (C) (APPROXIMATE)
250°F	120°C
300°F	150°C
325°F	165°C
350°F	180°C
375°F	190°C
400°F	200°C
425°F	220°C
450°F	230°C

WEIGHT

US STANDARD	METRIC (APPROXIMATE)
½ ounce	15 g
1 ounce	30 g
2 ounces	60 g
4 ounces	115 g
8 ounces	225 g
12 ounces	340 g
16 ounces or 1 pound	455 g

Other books by Karen Dixon:

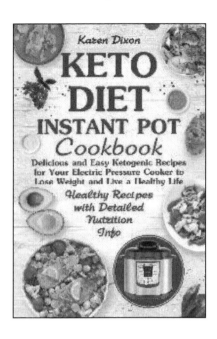

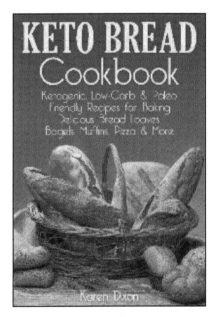

Made in the USA
Columbia, SC
23 July 2020

14558921R00078